HCG – DIET 2.0: LOSE WEIGT FAST AND FOREVER

EAT SMART AND LOSE WEIGHT WITHOUT STARVING

DAN HILD

ISBN 978-1-63957-042-3

Contents

ONE
HCG

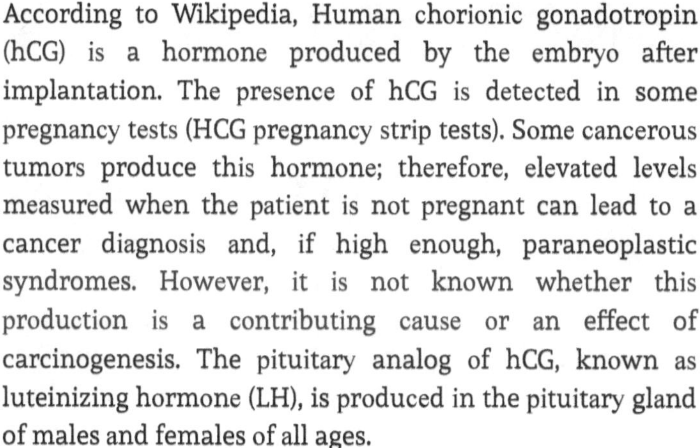

According to Wikipedia, Human chorionic gonadotropin (hCG) is a hormone produced by the embryo after implantation. The presence of hCG is detected in some pregnancy tests (HCG pregnancy strip tests). Some cancerous tumors produce this hormone; therefore, elevated levels measured when the patient is not pregnant can lead to a cancer diagnosis and, if high enough, paraneoplastic syndromes. However, it is not known whether this production is a contributing cause or an effect of carcinogenesis. The pituitary analog of hCG, known as luteinizing hormone (LH), is produced in the pituitary gland of males and females of all ages.

Regarding endogenous forms of hCG, there are various ways to categorize and measure them, including total hCG, C-terminal peptide total hCG, intact hCG, free β-subunit hCG, β-core fragment hCG, hyperglycosylated hCG, nicked hCG, alpha hCG, and pituitary hCG. Regarding pharmaceutical preparations of hCG from animal or synthetic sources, there are many gonadotropin preparations, some of which are medically justified and others of which are of a ?uack nature. As of December 6, 2011, the United States Food and Drug Administration has prohibited the sale of "homeopathic" and over-the-counter hCG diet products and declared them fraudulent and illegal.

HCG is a hormone secreted by the placenta during pregnancy (the same hormone detected in home pregnancy kits). It was first used to help weight loss because several physicians noted that overweight women actually lost weight when they were pregnant. More than a dozen medical studies have shown that combined with a low calorie diet and exercise, HCG increases fat loss and helps with loss of inches.

HCG has not been approved by the FDA for weight loss, although it has been approved for the treatment of other medical conditions. Federal laws allow medical providers to use approved drugs for alternative treatments. It is called "Off Label Usage" and occurs ?uite fre?uently in the medical profession.

HCG is used in extremely low doses for weight loss. Weekly injections of 20 units are recommended. More fre?uent injections may be given after re-evaluations and approval from your medical provider. HCG is used in a much higher dose (~140 times more than in daily injections) to increase fertility. In the small dose of 20 units, HCG does NOT increase fertility. However, fertility is increased with every five (5) pounds of weight loss! HCG can cause a false positive pregnancy test in urine only.

Some of the benefits of HCG include the following:

- Positive effect on mood
- Increased energy levels
- Relief of back pain
- Relief of migraine pain

- More rapid loss of inches

In the past, some patients have not qualified for our regular weight loss program. This has been due to them not being the recommended percentage over their ideal weight or their BMI being within the normal range. Since HCG affects only the abnormal fat, such as "belly fat" or the "spare tire," a larger number of patients will ?ualify for this treatment.

TWO

GENERAL INFORMATION

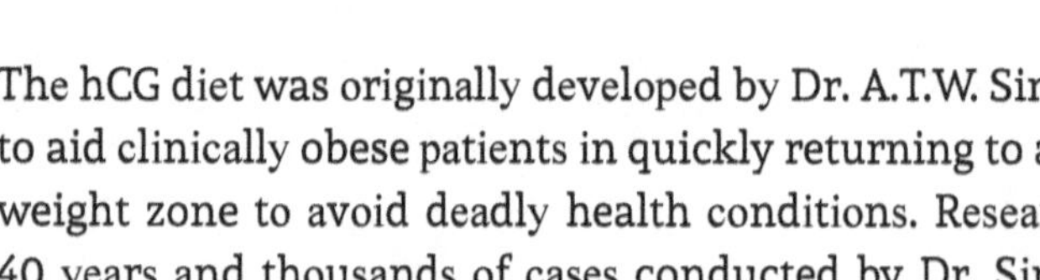

The hCG diet was originally developed by Dr. A.T.W. Simeons to aid clinically obese patients in quickly returning to a safer weight zone to avoid deadly health conditions. Research of 40 years and thousands of cases conducted by Dr. Simeons has lead to the concept of the hCG diet, which is meant to be a healthier interpretation and implementation of weight loss rather than the purely cosmetic, over-hyped diets of today. Unlike other mainstream diets, the hCG diet refocuses one's attention to smaller portions, less fatty foods, less fatty topical products and structured routines that promote more long-term weight-loss. It is not a diet solely for the purpose of losing weight to look good.

It is combined with rapid weight loss to help patients get back into safer weight zones so that they are out of immediate danger and can focus on the internal changes that will promote healthier living for years to come.

There are several variations and protocols of the original hCG diet. However, interpreted, the consumption of foods such as sweet fruits, starches, eggs and milk are carefully limited or omitted during the treatment process. The hCG diet also limits the use of certain topical products such as lotions, chapstick and conditioners which contain fatty substances and harmful chemicals that may react with or defeat the purpose of the hCG.

Dr. Simeons wrote a book called Pounds and Inches for other doctors and he states that HCG causes a change in metabolism. He states it makes your body mobilize fat out of the fat storage locations. Weight loss comes from adipose tissue, not muscle. And HCG does not strip the body of vitamins and minerals. And if you follow the diet, you can keep that weight off!

- Assists patients in shedding up to 30+ pounds over a 5-6 week period.
- Assists in the reduction of cholesterol and blood sugar levels.
- Dramatically reduces the appearance of cellulite.
- Results in the disappearance of food cravings.
- Increases energy levels.
- Decreases blood pressure.
- Improves skin elasticity
- Is safe and healthy.

How does it work?

The HCG diet consists of daily injections or oral drops of HCG. It is similar to what a diabetic person does when they inject insulin daily. The oral form is simply put into your mouth with a dropper. In addition to this, you will need to reduce your caloric intake to just 500 calories per day. Generally you eat a meal of lean meat, chicken, fish, shrimp or lobster, one fruit and one vegetable, two times a day. (There are a few exceptions.)

Obviously, you would be able to lose weight with a 500-calorie diet even if you weren't getting HCG hormone treatments. If you cut back to this many calories without the help of HCG, however, you will likely be very hungry and lose muscle as well as fat.

Obviously, this isn't healthy and will not result in a toned body.

What can I expect?

There are no age or sex limits, and tolerance to the treatment is excellent. Weight loss is safe and comfortable for patients, provided that they meticulously follow the prescribed diet. Any deviation from the protocol is likely to not yield the desired results. Even minor deviations may cause unwanted setbacks. At the conclusion of the diet patients should have lost an average of 0.5 - 1.0lb per day.

You will lose fat mostly in the waist and stomach. You'll reduce any fat pads like a double chin and love handles. You'll lose that inner knee and thigh fat with no sagging skin. The diet actually helps you do body contouring without exercise. HCG makes it easier for you to cut back calories because it acts as an appetite suppressant. During the first few days of the program, you might experience mild hunger after reducing your food consumption. By the second week, however, most people find small servings of food to be ?uite satisfying. This is partially because the HCG helps to release calories from your stored fat and these calories then circulate throughout your body. In addition, your hypothalamus makes adjustments to your metabolic rate, which helps you feel full faster.

Each person will have a different weight loss goal and the length of the program will be customized to meet his or her particular needs. Many patients willingly submit to a second or third treatment.

The HCG Diet is a physician supervised plan that will allow you to reach your weight loss goals in a shorter time frame than conventional "dieting." Clinically we find that balanced structured meals combined with daily use of HCG allow the body to tap into and metabolize its stored fat. This allows for a safe, rapid loss of fat and inches.

What happens to the body after years of dieting?

Diet programs can have good results if a change in lifestyle and eating habits is achieved.

How many of us have been on a diet, lost a good amount of weight, then gained it back? Most diets consist of reducing calories. After years of doing this, the body is in chaos and doesn't know what to do any more. This can slow your metabolism and affect your hormones. Pretty soon as another diet is introduced, the body will hold on to the fat and not let it go because it knows it's diet time again.

THREE

PREPARING FOR THE DIET

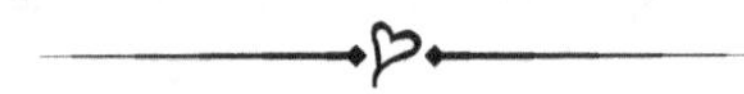

Mental Preparation:

Recognize the need to lose weight.

It is difficult to succeed in anything without a full understanding as to why you are doing it. Write down all the reasons as to why you are going to succeed with this diet. Remember, these goals are what will keep you committed and focused throughout the entire protocol.

Physical Preparation:

(1) Create an inventory of foods that conform to the hCG Diet.

Calculate the ?uantities that will be re?uired to get you through the entire hCG Diet protocol, be it a short protocol or the 40 day protocol. Create a grocery list if you do not have enough in your current inventory. Remember, to purchase the appropriate spices and sweeteners.(Stevia, Cayenne, Ground Pepper, Dill, Garlic, Ginger, Non-iodized salts, etc...)

(2) Prepare the first weeks meals ahead of time.

Cook the meats thoroughly and keep refrigerated. Some menu items will be fine kept frozen. Not being prepared will make the diet more difficult to stay committed to. We have multiple recipes submitted by various customers that we know to conform to the weight loss plan. By diversifying your menu you don't feel the desire to skip meals or cheat. The easiest way to set yourself up for failure is to not be prepared. Pre-cook 3 to 4 of your meals ahead of time. Grill your meats outside. If the weather doesn't cooperate, try an indoor grill like the George Foreman grill. Meat may also be sautéed in water or baked. The purpose in precooking (primarily your meats) is to be prepared. If you are in a rush it makes it easier to get stuck in a bind with nothing on hand but a convenience store, restaurant, or vending machine. Those foods are tempting enough, especially when first beginning a change in lifestyle. SO, be prepared. Most likely you won't gain cheating here and there but it will slow down the diet process for 1 to 3 days and for some people they lose enthusiasm and quit. Be prepared! Stay focused. It's a very small sacrifice.

The hCG diet is only days, not years long. It is short yet when done properly the weight stays off.

Fast food, vending machines and convenience stores won't prepare the foods as well as you will nor do most of their menu items conform to the hCG Diet.

(3) Know your goal and starting point.

Use charts to keep track of weight loss and inches lost. Monitor daily. Weigh yourself each morning after waking up and eliminating. Wear similar outfits to weigh yourself as each outfit may vary in weight. Keep your charts by the scale and near a mirror. We have found that for most people the first ten pounds lost are not noticeable. The following pounds will show significantly

as well as the measurements will show significant reduction in inches. Choose a day to start. **(STAY COMMITTED!)**

FOUR

THE PLAN

The HCG diet plan consists of 3 stages: The first 2 load days, the 500 calorie fat burning stage, and the maintenance diet.

Loading days:

Days 1 – 2:

Begin taking the HCG hormone as instructed. These are "loading days," which consist of eating as many fat filled foods as possible until you are completely stuffed. Dr. Bird suggests eating a lot of highly concentrated foods such as milk chocolate, pastries, sugar, fried meats, eggs and bacon, mayonnaise, bread with thick butter and jam etc.

The time and trouble spent on pressing this point upon reluctant patients is always greatly rewarded afterwards, because they do not struggle with the difficulties of hunger and fatigue in the beginning stages of the diet. Patients who do not follow instructions on the loading days have a much more difficult time in the beginning and have a more difficult first week.

500-calorie Fat Burning Stage:

Day 3 - until last dose of HCG:

Continue taking the prescribed dose of HCG. Begin the 500-calorie per day diet. This will be explained further below.

72 hours after last dose of HCG:

Transition stage - STOP taking the HCG:

Continue on the 500 calorie diet for 72 more hours. The hormone will be completely eliminated from the body.

The Maintenance Diet, weeks 1-3:

Begin 72 hours after your last dose of HCG and continue for three weeks. You may now eat more foods and add fats and dairy into your diet. NO starches or sugars are allowed in this phase. The purpose of this phase is for the body to adjust and stabilize at its new weight.

The Maintenance Diet, weeks 4-6:

This is the final phase where you begin to add starches and sugars back into your diet.

Technically nothing is off limits anymore. It is best not to resume any old eating habits that led to weight gain in the first place, but you may eat what you would like. The best rule to follow is "everything in moderation." More information about this will be provided.

Supplies needed:

- Scale to measure your weight. You need to weigh yourself every morning. This allows you to see your progress and identify any problems when there is no weight loss.
- Digital food scale that measures in ounces. Digital is preferred, because it is more accurate. Varying food weight, even if it is just an ounce, can affect your weight loss.

Important Points:

Weight Fluctuations

After the fourth or fifth day of dieting the daily loss of weight begins to decrease and there is a smaller urinary output. Men often continue to lose regularly at that rate, but women are more irregular in spite of faultless dieting. There may be no drop at all for two or three days and then a sudden loss, which reestablishes the normal average. These fluctuations are entirely due to variations in the retention and elimination of water, which are more common in women than in men.

Two processes determine the weight registered by the scale. Under the influence of HCG, fat is being extracted from the cells, in which it is stored in the fatty tissue. When these cells are empty and therefore serve no purpose, the body breaks down the cellular structure and absorbs it, but breaking up of useless cells, connective tissue, blood vessels, etc., may lag behind the process of fat-extraction. When this happens the body appears to replace some of the extracted fat with water, which is retained for this purpose. As water is heavier than fat the scales may show no loss of weight, although sufficient fat has actually been consumed to make up for the deficit in the 500-Calorie diet. When then such tissue is finally broken down, the water is liberated and there is a sudden flood of urine and a marked loss of weight. This simple interpretation of what is really an extremely complex mechanism is the one we give those patients who want to know why it is that on certain days they do not lose, though they have committed no dietary error.

Cosmetics

Skin care products with fats, oils, butters, creams and ointments can be absorbed and interfere with weight reduction by HCG just as if they have been eaten. This sensitivity to very minor increases in nutritional intake is a unique feature of the HCG diet. Anyone who handles fats, such a hair dressers, massage therapists, butchers, etc. never show a satisfactory loss of weight unless they can avoid fat coming into contact with their skin. Make sure to check any lotions or sunscreens for fats and oils before you use them. Lotions that are entirely free of fatty substances may be used with caution.

Otherwise, stick to only using mineral oil based products such as baby oil or baby night time/bedtime lotion for dry skin. You can also use Cornhuskers lotion, which is glycerin based. Glycerin attracts moisture to your skin, so it will soften you skin. There are glycerin-based soaps as well which can be used in the shower.

Make-up

Make-up that is allowed on the diet is: eye brow pencil, eyeliner, mascara, lipstick, and face powder that are oil-free. For those who cannot live without make-up, others

have used mineral make-up on the protocol without adverse affects on the ability to lose weight. If you currently are using mineral make -up, then you may continue to use it. If not, then we recommend Young Blood mineral make-up. Basically, mineral make-up is the best and only option.

Possible acne breakouts

It is possible to have acne outbreaks while on the protocol. Our fat cells are storage for everything, from vitamins and minerals to toxins. If you have an acne flare-up or rash occur during the diet, it is most likely your body's way of excreting toxins. Our skin is

a large detox organ, and when there are too many toxins for the liver to handle efficiently, then the skin will step in and excrete some of those toxins as well.

Shampoo/Conditioner

Most shampoo and conditioners are fine. If your conditioner has oils in it, you may either switch conditioners, or use the one you have as long as you rinse it out IMMEDIATELY after putting it on your hair. Do not let it sit on your hair and do not massage into your scalp. You may also want to check your deodorant; if it has oil in it you shouldn't use it. You can switch to some sort of deodorant spray while on the diet.

Mineral oil

Many women who are adjusted to the use of cosmetics and skin care products containing fat find that their skin gets dry as soon as they stop using them. Mineral oil may be used as a treatment for dry skin, because its molecules are too large to be absorbed by the skin.This point also creates controversy, because the oil becomes a layer over the skin and clogs pores. It is also a petroleum-based product that is a byproduct of refining oil. If this does not bother you, you can use mineral oil for dry skin, because the body will not absorb it. Mineral oil is able to keep skin moisturized, because it is an extra layer on top of the skin. Mineral oil should not be used in preparing the food, because of its laxative ?uality and the fact that it absorbs fat soluble vitamins, which are then lost in the stool.

Mineral oil scrub

Another way to use Mineral oil is to mix sea salt with baby oil to make a thick body scrub. The scrub will remove dead skin, leaving skin smooth and soft. Use it on the driest areas, such as elbows, knees, heels, etc. Rinse well after the scrub, in order to remove all residue. You may follow by washing the area with glycerin soap.

Menstruation

For women who menstruate no HCG injections are given during the monthly menstrual cycle. This is done for up to four days. If after four days the period is worse the patient needs to speak with the doctor. The 500-calorie diet is continued during menstruation and causes no hardship because HCG is still circulating in the body.

Vitamins

Every time you lose a pound of fatty tissue only the actual fat is burned up. All the vitamins, the proteins, the blood, and the minerals that this tissue contains in abundance are fed back into the body. If there are certain vitamins you need or want to take they need to be discussed with the doctor.

Salt and Reducing

There is no restriction in the use of salt but patients need to drink large quantities of water throughout the treatment. Your daily amount taken should be roughly the same or less, as a sudden increase in salt will of course be followed by a corresponding increase in water weight as shown by the scale. An increase in the intake of salt is one of the most common causes for an increase in weight from one day to the next.

Water

The amount of water you retain has nothing to do with the amount of water you drink. When the body is forced to retain water, it will do this at all costs. If water intake is insufficient, excessive water will be withdrawn from the intestinal tract, with the result of possible constipation. On the other hand if a patient drinks more than his body re?uires, the surplus is promptly and easily eliminated. Trying to prevent the body from retaining water by drinking less does not work. A 2-liter minimum should be consumed each day.

Constipation

Your bowel movements will slow down due to the decreased intake of food. If you drink the proper amount of water you can avoid constipation. If constipation does become an issue then speak with the doctor to get some ideas and suggestions.

Beginning days 1 & 2, the "loading days"

Administer the HCG as directed (injection or oral dose). Eat as much as you want, especially high fat. It is important to get the HCG into your system before you start the diet plan. Do NOT try to limit your food during these days; the fattening food is necessary for the diet to work correctly. The more you eat, the better results you will have. Those who do not load to the fullest also experience difficult hunger pains throughout the injections. It is also possible to gain weight on the loading days; you will lose it all within the first week, probably even the first 2 days! Don't worry! It may seem impossible to load yourself with really fatty, unhealthy items (especially if you're on your second or third round of the protocol.) Examples of healthier fats: Cold pressed oils, avocados, nuts/seeds, nut butters & tahini. Eat foods that your crave that are especially high in fat such as: ice cream, cakes, cookies, custards, creams, pastries, chocolate, etc. as it has a psychological effect of saying "good bye" (for now!)

FIVE
DAY 3

Continue HCG as directed. Begin the 500 calories per day plan. The 500-calorie limit per day MUST be maintained.

Breakfast: Water, tea, coffee in any amount "without" sugar. One tablespoon of milk is allowed in 24 hours. Stevia may be used to sweeten. Some people choose to have a small portion of fruit for their breakfast.

Lunch & Dinner: You are allowed one protein and one vegetable. A spreadsheet will be provided to you that will help plan your meals and make sure you are eating the correct amount of calories. You can choose to use it or not. As mentioned previously, a safe way to divide up the 500 calories is allotting 300 calories towards protein, 120 calories towards fruit, and 80 calories towards vegetables. This is only a guideline and it doesn't have to be exact. For those people who want to keep this diet as simple as possible there is another way to set it up so that things are much easier. See the following table:

The HCG Diet Weight Loss Protocol

- Phase 1: Day 1 & 2, Two LOAD days! Begin your HCG drops. Take 10 drops (up to 20 drops) of HCG 3-times a day under your tongue and hold for at least 15 seconds before swallowing. Wait 30 minutes before eating, 1 hr before caffeine, coffee, tea or Zevia (cola). On these days eat as much as you can of high fat foods.

Remember focus on FATS instead of sugars. Be in a constant state of "stuffed" for 2 days. This Phase is crucial, because unless your normal fat reserves are well-stocked, you will not remain comfortably on the 500 calorie diet. You will gain a few pounds these first two days. However it will promptly come off. So ENJOY the ice cream and cheese cake!!

- Phase 2: Day 3—23 (up to 43 days), Now watch the weight come off. Continue your drops as above and begin the 500 calorie diet. It is important and desirable that you include some B-Vitamins while on this low calorie diet. Vitamins B-6 and B-12 have been conveniently and economically added to the HCG Weight Loss Formula. Begin the very low calorie diet (500 calories outlined below). Stay on this until you have completed the HCG diet. You must continue the 500 calorie diet for three days after your last drops. This is a very essential part of the protocol because, HCG remains in your system for up to 3 days; working for you. If you start eating normally, as long as there is even a trace of HCG in your system, you could put on weight. After three days, when all the HCG, has been eliminated, you can begin phase 3.

- Phase 3: Three Week Maintenance Phase (21 days): You must avoid all sugars or starches for 3 weeks. This is very critical because this is when your body resets your metabolism and hypothalamus for your new body weight. It takes about 3 weeks after following this protocol to become stable. Your calories should be a minimum of 1500 a day. This is a perfect time to add exercise back into your schedule. The goal here is to stay stay within 2-3 pounds above or below the last weight you recorded while still taking HCG. If you exceed the 2 -3 pounds, you should do a "Steak Day" to take off the extra weight. Steak Day: eat nothing for breakfast and lunch and have a large steak and apple or steak and tomato for dinner that night. Drink lots of water. Your weight will be back down the following day. If you lose more than 2 pounds from your last recorded weight while on HCG, you aren't eating enough. Please note that people, who gain their weight back, usually failed at this part of the diet. So be STRICT with yourself...IT IS WORTH IT!!

- Phase 4: Enjoy the person you are meant to be! Slowly introduce sugar and healthy carbs back into your diet in small amounts while keeping a close eye on the scale. Remember your "Steak Day" if you get 2-3 pounds over your last recorded weight while you were still taking your hCG drops.

Stalls, Gains, and Fluctuations:

This protocol must be followed exactly as described. The slightest deviation from our recommendations could affect your ability to lose weight and is immediately detectable at the daily weighing. Pay attention to weight gains; they usually signify an error in the protocol.

Keep a detailed food journal and look for patterns of foods that cause you not to lose, or to lose fantastically. Some people have had problems losing with tomatoes and oranges (but some people have no problem at all). Since everyone is different, you need to monitor your own body and see what works or doesn't work for you.

Eating too many calories or foods not on your list can cause problems. Weight gains/stalls may take a few days to kick in. For example, you could mix your veggies for a few days and assume there is no problem based on what the scale reads, but then a stall or gain can suddenly reflect the breaking of the rules. Many people believe a stall comes out of nowhere, but it is usually caused by something.

If more salt is eaten in the food you prepare and your body isn't used to that sodium level, your blood volume will increase to handle the extra, which will translate into a gain because your body is retaining water to boost that blood volume. Watch your salt intake.

Sensitivity / allergies to foods may cause weight stalls. Listen to your body.

Not drinking enough water: Must drink half of your body weight in ounces. Also be aware that many things contain sugar or fats that we may not realize as: chewing gum, mints, vitamins, cough syrups, etc.........

Plateau: This can occur with anyone and can last 4-6 days. If you lose more than the average you may plateau sooner. The plateau always corrects itself and should not cause you to worry. If however you wish to break up the plateau after three days it is permissible to do an apple day. An apple day consists of only eating 6 apples while drinking your normal-fluids. No other types of food are eaten during this day. You should see a 1 2lb weight loss the next morning.

A Mini Steak Day is also option when weight is stalled and no hunger is present.

- Drink allowable drinks all day
- Have a 3.5oz. steak with an apple for dinner
- Following day return to the normal 500 calorie diet

Menstrual period: Weight loss slows down a few days before and during the menstrual cycle and for some women at the time of ovulation. In women, menstrual periods can increase water retention, and water weight shows on the scale. If you know you are following the plan and are not, you just need to accept that the stall / gain is temporary and continue to follow protocol. The drop will happen once the menstrual cycle is normalized in the body. The best time to begin the injections is right after finishing your period but if this is not possible the minimum of 8-10 injections are needed before onset. During the first 4 days of the menstrual cycle no injections are taken but 500-calorie diet is maintained. After the 4 days injections are resumed. If your period only lasts three days then the injections are not done for those 3 days.

Cosmetics: Use of lotions, face creams, soaps etc.... all can contribute to stalls in weight loss. All beauty care products that contain oils are to be discontinued except for glycerin and mineral oil based products. Shampoo and conditioner are OK to use providing they are washed out quickly.

It is important to know that what works for one person does NOT mean it will work for everyone; to prevent stalls / gains simply do not make changes to this protocol just because someone else is losing with that modification. This is especially important when researching recipes, always check ingredients against the diet plan provided for you.

Tips and Hints for the 500-calorie diet

This is a protocol of not just food, but mental preparation as well. This also involves planning of how you are going to handle the day-to-day situations that will derail you, the roadblocks you may come across, and how you are going to handle them. People will ask you ?uestions, be prepared to plan your meals...etc

Take the time to memorize the protocol and make sure your schedule is ready to take on your new diet. Spend time planning your meals and shopping for the foods allowed on the protocol.

In the beginning it is best not to totally rely on your memory and check every meal against the diet list before starting to eat. Keep a food diary with everything you eat and the times it was consumed. Include your morning weight and how much was lost from the day before.

Track your li?uids (variety and amount). Try to keep a running account of calories so you ensure your remain within the 500 calories.

Since you will be eating many of the same things, it is great to buy and cook your meat portions in advance. It saves time in the long run and helps you stick to the diet.

It's great idea to keep a few "snacks" readily available for when a craving hits:

- Slice up an apple and mix Stevia with cinnamon and dip the apple slices.
- Create a strawberry smoothie: ice water, strawberries, stevia (optional), lemon juice (optional).
- Crunchy snack: celery sticks OR cucumbers
- For the fast meal: precook some chicken (weigh your portions first) and wash and dry full heads of lettuce, store these in the refrigerator. These preparations ahead of time allow you to prepare a quick dinner of chicken salad. Make a dressing out of lemon, apple cider vinegar and fresh pepper. This is great when you want an enormous portion, it's difficult to eat too much lettuce (low calories).
- Don't be afraid of hunger because hunger is a feeling (physical sensation) not a fact.

- Remember that the HCG is providing more than enough fat and nutrients to meet your needs.

When hunger strikes:

- Drink 2 big glasses of water
- Space your meals throughout the day so you are constantly eating

- You can have coffee/tea in the morning when you wake-up (8:00am) o Eat an apple at mid-morning (10:00am)
- Have a grissini/melba toast in the early afternoon (12:00) o Eat your lunch mid afternoon (2:00)
- Eat your second grissini late afternoon (4:00) o Eat dinner in the evening (6:00)

- Your second fruit in the late evening (8:00)
- Coffee and teas tend to curb your appetite
- Phentermine is a prescribed appetite suppressant many choose to use during the diet. You can speak with your doctor about this if it has not already been prescribed to you.
- Hoodia is an herbal suppressant that is available for those who wish not to take phentermine, or are not able to take phentermine. You can speak to your physician about this.
- You can be prepared and make teas for the week. Some teas to use are Yerba
- Mate, Chaior Chocolate, Oolong, Chamomile, Green tea, (these are all organic). Put a gallon of spring water in a large pot and use 3 – 5 teabags and a few drops of Stevia. Allow it to sit for a while to cool off then move it to the refrigerator.

- Label each tea if you make more than one tea at a time.
- If you cannot live without soda, make your own using sparkling water and flavored Stevia. DO NOT drink Diet sodas as they contain Aspartame.
- Be precise in your counting of calories and weighing of food. One tenth of an ounce can make a big difference.
- To create ground beef (do not buy from the store ... this is too fatty and not allowed): ask the butcher to trim all the fat from a lean piece of steak, ask him to show it to you after he/she trims (to be sure it is suitable for you), and then ask to have it ground. You can also do this at home by trimming the fat off of the meat, cutting it into cubes, and placing it in a food processor or blender.
- If you have difficulty finding a small apple, you can just cut a large one in half and only eat half. You can also use thins method for oranges. This will also help you save calories (especially good for beef days).
- Muscle Fatigue: Sometimes, at the end of a full course, when a lot of fat has been rapidly lost, some patients complain that lifting a weight or climbing stairs re?uires a greater muscular effort than before. This is caused by the removal of abnormal fat deposited between, in, and around the muscles, and disappears soon after the end of the treatment. Taking potassium 99mg per day may help this, but if it does not, reassure yourself that your strength will return soon after the diet has ended.
- Massage: For those who seek to do massage therapy purely for muscle aches and cramping, you must use mineral oil, there are no other options. Massage is typically not recommended while on the HCG diet due to hypersensitivity of tissues.

Tips on Managing Cheating:

- Do not be afraid of cheating. You always have complete control whether you give into temptation or not. Just because someone else has cheated does not mean you will cheat as well. Many, many people have followed this plan without cheating, and you can too. Prepare yourself for the fact that you will *want* to cheat, but *acting* on the thought is solely your decision.
- Expect to have cravings, be hungry, and moody and expect to want to cheat.
- These expectations will let you be prepared to control the cravings, hunger, moods and cheats. Prepare yourself for these feelings, but know that the decision to deviate is yours...........stay strong and remember that only you are accountable for everything you put into your mouth.
- If you go forward and cheat, you will have to take responsibility for that cheat. It may leave you feeling guilty and unsatisfied. Cheating (even what may be perceived as just a small slip-up) is a mistake you will pay for up to 3-5 days. This can be 3 -5 days of the scale going up, or staying the same, potentially you could even gain more than if you were not on HCG. This makes cheating on this plan a

waste of time and money.... NOT WORTH IT!

- If you use food as an emotional crutch, you will find it difficult to cope without hat crutch while on the 500 calories. You need to fill the empty spot with something healthy that you can enjoy both on and off the protocol. This will not only reduce cravings, but also help you maintain your healthy weight into the future. Some possibilities include crafting, painting, walking, gardening, reading, visiting with friends (encourage friends to be creative and find activities to enjoy together that do not revolve around food)
- Create a cabinet in your kitchen and a designated shelf in your fridge which supports your diet.
- To get your mind off of wanting to cheat, focus your attention on something else.
- You can: take a walk, go to the library, go to a movie, visit with friends, brush your teeth, clean a closet, read a book, etc....
- It is also nice to find a support system, whether it is through an online group, a buddy who is following the diet with you, family member(s), etc. Join our weekly/ biweekly ?uestion and answer sessions for those following this plan. Just make sure you have someone to stop you from cheating.

Tips to Treat Ailments:

- Headache: Typically, an "aspirin" is okay. Some people have successfully used Excedrin, Advil, and Tylenol without any effects on weight loss. Just make sure to avoid the ones that have the shiny coating that makes them look like M&Ms!! That coating has sugar in it. We have successfully used both Ibuprofen and aspirin on the diet without any adverse effects on weight loss.
- Heartburn/Bloating: Take 1 Tablespoon full of apple cider vinegar, it should ease the acidic feeling.
- Sore Throat: Gargle with warm salt water
- Rash: Dilute apple cider vinegar with water in a 1:4 ratio. Use a washcloth and apply the solution directly on the rash. You may also use the Aveeno oatmeal bath soak to relieve itchiness of the rash. It is always best to leave the rash open anyways to allow it to "breathe" as it heals.
- Stressful situations: Bach Rescue Remedy drops or spray (found at Whole Foods or Sprouts) for a calming effect.
- Constipation: Smooth Move Tea by Traditional Medicinals (found at Whole Foods or Sprouts). Make sure you are drinking the recommended amount of water each day

- Muscle Weakness/ Muscle Cramps: Potassium 99mg (1 cap) 2x per day.
- Leg Cramps: These during sleep are not uncommon and can be fre?uent and painful for those who experience them. To decrease or avoid them, asparagus can be decreased / avoided (it is a natural diuretic that may contribute to low potassium). Intake of spinach or chard can be increased as these vegetables are high in potassium. Increasing your daily dose of potassium can help with this as well.
- If you don't feel like eating, make sure you at LEAST eat small portions of proteins and the two fruits (these have high calories than the veggies).

Exercise:

· Importance of not doing a lot – doing a lot of exercise could hinder weight loss. When you build muscle, the muscle surrounds itself with water to heal and build.

This can cause temporary weight gain, and also interfere with weight loss. It is best to just do mild exercising while on the diet, and begin with more strenuous exercise in the stabilization phase.

· Walking, mild swimming, zero resistance biking – generally 30 -45 minutes 3 times a week is sufficient.

SIX

WEIGHT STABILIZATION

<u>Duration: This phase is 3-6 weeks</u>

- Importance: This phase involves stabilizing your body's metabolism at your new weight. This phase is just as important as the Fat Burning phase. You want to reset your metabolism at your new weight, so that your body does not fluctuate up or down on the scale. If you still need to lose more weight you may do a second round of HCG after this phase is completed.
- You must weigh yourself every morning as soon as you rise, but after you have urinated.
- Eat three meals a day. You may increase your meals in size and ?uantity, as long as you follow the rules below.

- Eat an adequate amount of daily calories to maintain weight.

ALL STARCHES AND SUGARS ARE AVOIDED FOR FIRST 3 WEEKS!!!!!

Avoid: sugar, breads, pastas, starchy vegetables (all potatoes, corn, dense s?uashes, carrots, and beets), rice, wheat, cereals, noodles, barley, any kind of flour, rye, food starch, etc. Beware of processed foods, because many will contain starches and sugars.

- Add in other veggies, and you may eat a variety of veggies in the same meal.
- Add in other fruits, except very sugary fruits (bananas, grapes, and any dried fruits).
- Add in fats and dairy products. Avocados, nuts, olive oils, good fats (like fatty fish), butter, cheese, and so on can be eaten at any meal.

Supplements: During this stage supplements are added in. Now that you are not burning your body's fat cells with stored nutrients, you need to supply your body with vitamins and minerals to function properly.

- EFA's – essential fatty acids (EFA's) are necessary for many functions in our bodies. They support everything from our skin and hair to our brain; our body needs a certain amount each and every day. If you do not eat the right amount per day, your body will cause you to crave fatty foods until you have met your body's needs Taking a supplement is an easy way to meet your body's needs, and to help curb unnecessary cravings for fatty foods.

- Multivitamin – a multivitamin will provide you with a portion of all of the
- vitamins and minerals you need for a healthy body. The food we eat may not contain the right amounts of vitamins and minerals, and it is always a good to supplement with a multivitamin.
- Enzymes – digestive enzymes help to break down food we eat. They can aid in digesting food, and help our bodies readjust to food we have not eaten for awhile.
- Keep in mind; you have been on a 500-calorie diet for weeks now. Do NOT go crazy and start eating 2500 calories on the 1st day after. Sneak up to it. Here is an example.
- First, find out your calorie limit: Women, this e?uates to 11 times your current weight, Men 12 times your current weight.
- Example: For a woman whose current weight is 150 lbs, multiplied times 11 is 1650 calories a day.
- Example: for a man whose current weight is 200, multiplied times 12 is 2400 calories a day.

Week 1- OK, so for week 1 after your 500 calorie diet, work your way up to about 800 -1000 calories a day. Remember no sugar, starches and low carbohydrates. Yes, you can eat fats during this time, but don't overdo it.

- Continue to drink lots of water. You can now eat 3+ meals a day.
- You can use butter, oil or cooking spray in your frying pan, just use it sparingly!
- Your protein will intake will increase to about 6-8 oz per meal or up to 600 calories per day. Your salad can now be a mixture of all your favorite things that you want in the salad, just no sugars, and starches.
- Try to eat a little at each meal and try to get in a mid morning and mid afternoon snack.

Week 2- Then for week 2, increase your daily calorie count to about 1000-1500 calories per day. Do this by adding in more veggies. Maybe some soups, cheese, peanut butter, nuts and other low carbohydrate type foods.

Week 3- Then by week 3 you can work your way up to your total calorie limit. You should be eating 5 or 6 little meals a day. Eat breakfast, a mid morning snack, Lunch, a mid-afternoon snack and Dinner. You might get away with a light dinner snack. Weight yourself every day and do not allow for more than a 2-pound gain. If there is, do a Steak day! This means skip breakfast and lunch on that day. At dinner, you are to eat a large steak an apple or a raw tomato. You may drink as much water as possible throughout the day.

The next day when you wake up, weigh yourself, and you should have dropped back down by at least 1 pound. Make sure you are weighing every day from the beginning of this phase. We cannot stress the importance of this. Many people think that they do not need to weigh themselves every day, and that they will be able to notice any weight gain. This is not necessarily true. Even if you are traveling, you need to take a scale with your and weigh yourself every morning to ensure you stabilize your weight.

Now, to add in the starches and sugars

Sugars and Starches (the carbohydrates) are the danger zone! Reintroduce these too fast, and you may have a weight gain. So to avoid that, this is what we have learned.

ADD them SLOWLY!

Week 4- So, for week 4 after your 500-calorie diet, add in the one carbohydrate food that you missed the most. Eat bread, pasta, potato or whatever, but just one. Then, the next day, stop that one and add another one. Do not eat two carb foods in the same day during week 4. Only eat one carb food per meal. Just change your carbohydrate from day to day. Weigh yourself the next day and see if there are any weight changes. If so, try cutting the portion in half for the next time.

Week 5- For week 5, combine 2 carb foods in the same day, but not at the same meal. Eat Bread with a sandwich for lunch and a potato for dinner or what

Week 6- For week 6, start combing the carbs during the same meal, but do this 1-day at a time. By the end of week 6, you should be eating a good, healthy, well rounded, high fiber, lower fat, diet within your calorie limit without worrying about gaining weight!

Avoid over-eating;(stay within your calorie limit) avoid eating both a high fat and high carb meal. You may get away with a high fat meal or a high carb meal but high fat and high carb together are a bad combination.

The Healthy Lifestyle

Portion control guidelines:

- Measuring portions when eating regular meals – This is a habit you will have developed during the HCG diet, and it is a good one to keep. You do not need to be fanatical about measuring, but this will help you gauge how much food you are actually eating. You will become accustom to looking at food and know the portion size, and this will help you when you eat at restaurants. So many times restaurant portions are so large, that we do not realize we are probably eating 2 and . meals at one sitting.
- Eating until the hunger sensation is gone, not until the "stuffed" sensation occurs

this is a problem many people have. It takes about 30 minutes for the satiety sensation (the sensation of being full) to set in after you have eaten a meal. If you eat till you feel completely full, you have overstuffed yourself. Eat normal size portions and watch your caloric intake, and you will be able to be full without feeling like a stuffed pig.

- "Eating to live, not living to eat." – this is the best advice I can give you. If you can begin to look at food as necessary fuel for your body instead of a treat, it will help you make the right choices. You will choose nutrient rich foods that will nourish your body over foods that are only made to satisfy the taste buds.

- Don't be afraid to indulge – Now, I say this with the greatest caution. Some people can go to a birthday party and have only once slice of cake with a little ice cream without craving more later. Others will have non-stop cravings once thy have tasted their favorite food again. My suggestion is that if you can control yourself, don't be afraid to eat ice cream, pizza, or whatever else you like, but not on a regular basis. If you are one of those people that cannot stop once you have tasted it, then do your best to stay away from trigger foods. Maybe find something else to indulge in every now and then that you know you will not crave. This diet is wonderful, because it will break you of any old habits that led to your weight gain, and you don't not want to reintroduce those habits again.

Healthy eating guidelines:

- Balance of nutrients: A healthy diet includes proteins, fats and carbohydrates. A healthy diet also includes veggies, fruits, grains (unless allergic), some sort of protein source (meat, soy, eggs, legumes, nuts etc.) fats, and ade?uate nutrients (such as vitamins and minerals).
- Cutting out any of the food groups can leave you unbalanced and unhealthy.
- Whole foods should be included in every diet: Foods in their natural form from the earth (i.e. veggies, fruits, unprocessed meats, and whole grains).
- Avoid any known food allergies. If you are unsure if you have any, we can run lab work to help you find out.

Protein:

- "Variety is the spice of life" - By this I mean eat a variety of protein sources, such as meat, chicken, beans, nuts, legumes, fish, eggs, soy, and dairy. This will allow you to rotate through food, and not eat the same thing every day.
- Meat: this includes beef, chicken, turkey, pork, and most other animal sources
- (excluding fish). Game meat and/or organically grown meat are the BEST meat to eat on a regular basis. You can find organic ranchers selling organic

buffalo, venison, chicken, beef, ostrich, lamb, and pork on the Internet at cheaper prices than in stores. Try to steer clear of / reduce your intake of processed meat products such as hot dogs, sausage, pepperoni, bacon, bologna, salami, and beef jerky. It is always best to eat whole foods, such as choosing steak or chicken over hot dogs and beef jerky. Also, the lower fat choices of meat are preferable, as beef is high in saturated fat. You can find cuts of beef that are lower in fat, or choose another alternative such as poultry (without the skin).

- Nuts: It is best to eat peanuts that are roasted, but all other nuts are more nutritious in their raw form. It is OK to eat roasted nuts, but the raw nuts are a better choice. Trader Joe's has one of the best selections for raw nuts at an affordable price. There are many types of nuts / seeds to choose from: walnuts, sunflower seeds, pumpkin seeds, cashews, pecans, filberts, almonds, brazil etc.

- Nut Butters: The best choice for nut butters is almond butter, cashew butter, and tahini. If you choose peanut butter, it is important that you get a good peanut butter with no added sugar or partially hydrogenated oils. Almost every grocery store sells these kinds of peanut butter. It is usually referred to as natural, but

- CHECK the INGREDIENTS. In natural peanut butters, the oil separates, so you have to mix it before using it. It helps if you store these in the fridge; that way the oil will naturally be mixed in with the nut butter and not sit on top (of course you have to mix it first before sticking it in the fridge).

- Beans, peas, and lentils: These are a great source of protein and fiber at the same time. There are many different ways to eat beans and lentils in order to satisfy any taste bud. If you have trouble digesting beans, then use BEANO or digestive enzymes as bean digestive aids. If you have not had much experience with beans in your diet and fear the gas effects of beans, these are a few things you can do to reduce such effects: Soak the beans in water overnight, then throw that water out and use new water to cook them in; in the beginning, cook beans one type at a time, so you can learn which ones you can tolerate well and which ones produce excessive gas. Every person is different in his / her bean tolerance.

- Fish: Avoid FARMED FISH if at all possible. Oily fish are the best to eat; 2 – 3 times a week is ideal. Some examples are salmon, herring, cod, trout, sardines, and halibut. You can also eat canned fish, but try to avoid tuna and make sure salmon is wild caught (check the can for wild caught Alaskan salmon). Farmed salmon is referred to as "Atlantic Salmon" and contains high amounts of toxins. It also has less health benefits. If you cannot afford or find wild caught salmon, then choose another fish. The healthiest cooking options for fresh fish are broiling, baking, and grilling. Fish with high environmental toxin contents are tuna steaks, mackerel, catfish, sturgeon, swordfish, and shark. These fish should be avoided. All fish are a bit contaminated, but some more than others. Other fish options are perch, red snapper, orange roughy, and tilapia. They do not contain good oils in them, but they do not have a high content of toxins, so they are OK to eat. Shrimp, clams, mussels, crab, lobster and so forth are also OK to eat.

- Eggs: Eggs are an excellent source of protein. One extra large egg had 8 gm of protein and one medium egg has 6gm of protein. Eggs are labeled in many different ways. The twp main things you want to look for are "organic" and "free range". Another label to look for is "Omega-3," but the first two are more important. Most supermarkets these days will have these types of eggs available.

- Supposedly healthier ways to cook eggs, if you are concerned about cardiovascular disease, are soft-boiled, sunny side up, or poached. However, I would not be too concerned with cooking methods as long as you are not frying or adding unhealthy ingredients.
- Soy: Soy products can help protect against breast cancer, prostate cancer, balance out female hormones, and lower cholesterol. Soy can lower the functioning of the thyroid; so if you have a thyroid condition, do not use this as your main source of protein. In general, I would not suggest overdoing soy. A good rule to live by is,
- Everything in Moderation." There are different types of soy:

a. **Tofu**(firm or baked), tempeh, miso soup. Buying firm or baked tofu and slicing and dicing and adding to recipes (soups, stir fries, casseroles, lasagnas, etc.) are an easy way to go. There are many different types of cookbooks out there with recipes to try as well.

b. **Soy meat analogs:** soy hotdogs, soy sausage, soy bologna, soy pepperoni, canadian bacon, soy burgers, and soy bacon. I do not recommend eating this type of soy on a regular basis, but it is a good substitute every now and then.

c. c. **Soy dairy alternatives:**UNSWEETENED soymilk, soy cheese, soy yogurt, soy ice cream and soy sour cream.

Many soymilks can be very high in sugar, so check your ingredients.

d. **Roasted soy nuts and Edamame:**(cooked soybeans ready to eat). These are great to have as a snack.

e. e. Soy Nut Butter

- Dairy: Dairy is a fine source of protein if you do not have any digestive issues with it. I would not suggest this to be your primary source of protein. The first and main rule with dairy is CHOOSE ORGANIC. Regular dairy products contain pesticides, added hormones, and antibiotics. I have found that changing to organic dairy versus regular will alleviate digestive problems for some people. If you can only afford some things as organic in your diet, dairy should be near the top of your list. Almost all grocery stores carry organic milk. The second rule of dairy is: DO NOT EAT ARTIFICIAL CHEESES (Velveeta, Pasteurized Process Cheese Foods, and American cheese. They contain very little nutritional value, and there are so many other better options for cheese.

- For Cheese, it is best to buy low fat (made with some skim milk). Farmer's Cheese and Ricotta cheese are two good choices because they are naturally low in fat.
- For Milk, you can use skim milk, or the lowest fat milk you can.

- For Yogurt, it is best to use PLAIN and add your own fruit. All fruited yogurts contain high amounts of sugar, even if they are organic. Use Stevia to sweeten the yogurt.
- Creams of all kinds should usually be avoided, due to the high saturated fat and caloric content. It is OK to use them every now and then, but do not use this as a staple in your diet. You will also need to watch out for cream soups and alfredo sauces, because they use cream as a main ingredient. Choosing light sauces or vegetable based sauces (tomato) is a better alternative to cream based sauces.

- Eat the proteins that work best with your body and digestion. If you are unsure which ones they are, then keep a diet diary to evaluate any digestive symptoms you may have (bloating, gas, constipation, diarrhea, heart burn, etc.)
- Protein intake should be at least 0.8gm/kg. One pound = 2.2kg, so divide your weight by 2.2 and then multiply it by 0.8 to find out how much protein you need per day. Most people think they need a lot more protein than they actually do.
- You should calculate how much you need for your body, and add in more if you are doing heavy weight lifting or training for something, such as a marathon.

Fats:

- Good oils should be a fundamental part of any diet. They contain essential nutrients in them that are a necessity for us to be healthy (Omega-3 and Omega-6 oils). There are also oils we need to avoid entirely that can be damaging to our bodies. Neutral oils, found in dairy and fat, are OK in moderation only.

- Bad Oils – AVOID Partially Hydrogenated Oils (PHOs), otherwise known as trans fat (trans fatty acid), Vegetable Fat, and Vegetable Shortening. This type of oil is added to a large amount of processed food, and is VERY UNHEALTHY TO EAT. You must READ your labels, and do not buy food with this in it.

Examples of foods with PHOs in regular grocery stores are: margarines, and other fake butter products, Crisco/shortenings, cookies, crackers, peanut butter, candy, pastries/muffins, butter-flavored microwave popcorn, Cool Whip, potato chips, tortilla chips, non-dairy creamers, and basically most frozen and prepared foods.

At health food stores or health aisles in grocery stores, you can find most of the above foods without the PHOs in them. PHOs are what make certain foods bad, and the foods themselves are not bad. Other oils on a label besides PHOs are fine.

- Good Oils – Butter (organic), extra virgin olive oil, Flax seed oil (do not cook with it, but it can be added to salads), Coconut oil, and unrefined, high oleic safflower oil (if it does not say those words on the label, then it is not the right kind of oil). If you cannot have dairy, you can buy Earth Balance instead of butter and margarine. DO NOT EAT SOY MARGARINE!!
- Essential fatty acids: Your body needs a daily amount of essential fatty acids (EFAs, otherwise known as Omega-6s and Omega-3s). Oily fish are a good way to consume these (salmon, sardines, etc) and flax seed oil is high in EFAs.

Most people need to supplement with EFAs on a regular basis (as discussed in Phase 2.

- If you do not meet your daily needs, your body will continue to crave large amounts of fatty foods (like chocolate, ice-cream, and fried foods).
- Monounsaturated fats: There are three kinds of fat in food – saturated, polyunsaturated, and monounsaturated oils. Good places to find Monounsaturated oils are olive oil, avocados, nuts (almonds and hazelnuts) and seeds (sesame seeds and pumpkin seeds). It is best to cook with oils that are monounsaturated, because they have the highest oxidation threshold; i.e. they remain stable at higher temperatures and do not easily become hydrogenated or saturated.

Grains:

- The first rule of grain is always use WHOLE GRAINS. Whole grain options are 100% whole wheat or other grain bread, brown and wild rice, and any whole grain product (crackers/pasta/pancakes/muffins, whole wheat bagels, etc.) Numerous stores have whole grain mixes for muffins, pancakes, waffles and more.
- Wheat is a widespread food allergen, so try to limit this in your diet. It is ideal to limit wheat intake to once or twice a week, but this is difficult for most people. I suggest limiting wheat to one serving per day, and using other grains/beans/lentils as alternative sources for carbohydrate and fiber intake. Other grain options are: oats, spelt, millet, barley, rye, corn, amaranth, quinoa, teff and rice. Remember, "Everything in moderation" and "Variety is the spice of life."

- Cereals: For Hot cereal, any unsweetened one is good. Choices are oatmeal and cream of rye/rice/wheat. Do NOT use sweetened instant packets. You may add fruit and Stevia to make great flavors for hot cereal (such as fresh berries and vanilla cream Stevia to oatmeal). For cold cereals, there are many options of healthy cereals at health food stores and healthy aisles at supermarkets. Plain Grape Nuts, Perky's Nutty Rice, and Unfrosted Shredded Wheat are the only regular cereals that are whole grain, sugar free and don't have any partially hydrogenated oils (see oil section for explanation).
- Crackers: Buy whole grain crackers without partially hydrogenated oils. Other options are Plain Rye-Krisp/ Rye-Vita, WASA, Ak-Maks, rice and popcorn cakes. For rice cakes, Hains/Health Valley brands are good, but eat only the plain variety in the Quaker Oats brand.
- Avoid any known food allergies.

Veggies:

- It is IMPORTANT to eat at least 5 – 9 servings of vegetables everyday (a serving is a cup). Fresh or frozen vegetables can be used, although fresh have more nutrients. Avoid canned vegetables, because they have no nutritional value and may have added sugars. If you boil vegetables, it will decrease their nutritional value (it's OK sometimes, but do not only eat boiled vegetables). Better lettuce options versus Iceberg lettuce are: red or green leaf, romaine, spinach, kale, cabbage, collard greens, beet greens, mustard greens, etc. A good rule of thumb is "The darker the green the better." Eating raw veggies is best, for they contain the highest amount of nutrients and enzymes. If you have problems digesting raw veggies, then cook before you eat. Good cooking options are: stir fry, steam, or bake them. An easy way to add veggies into a diet is to add vegetables to your sandwich at lunch, eating a baked potato or half a s?uash and some cooked veggies at dinner, and snacking on carrots, celery, or cherry tomatoes. You can also shred or grind up veggies and add them to sauces to get kids to eat veggies they hate. Vegetables are also a source of fiber, so increasing veggie intake increases fiber in your diet.

- Cruciferous family vegetables are a nourishing vegetable choice. Examples are: (broccoli, cauliflower, brussel sprouts, radish, cabbage, onions, and garlic. Colors are good: mix up your veggie colors by including orange, yellows, greens, and purples, because different colors contain different vitamins and minerals. Many green options have been listed already. Good orange veggie choices are: carrots, s?uash, yams, and sweet potatoes. Remember, everything in moderation. ALL veggies have their value and you should strive both for fre?uency of intake and diversity.

- Salads are a good way to get fresh vegetables into your diet. You can make them interesting and different, so you don't get bored with the same old salad every day. Good salad additions to spice up the flavor are pickles, olives, sunflower seeds, raisins, dried cranberries, fresh strawberries, grated cheese, and raw nuts. The ideal choices for salad dressings are olive oil or flax seed oil with vinegar (balsamic is s great choice) or lemon juice, Italian, Caesar, and different vinaigrette dressings. Personally, I like the brand called "Annie's" There are a variety of choices for flavors and most do not have added sugar or bad oils. You can find these in the healthy aisles at grocery stores, Trader Joe's, Whole Foods, Wild Oats, Sprouts, and Henry's Market. Another great brand is Spectrum at Fry's Marketplace (Smith's) grocery stores (in the healthy food aisles). Avoid heavy dressings like blue cheese, thousand island, and Fat Free dressings. If you are choosing healthy brands of dressings, then the fat in them is good fat (see oils section for more explanation.)

Fruits:

- Fruit intake should be one or two pieces a day. Eat fresh fruit versus juices, dried fruits, canned fruit, etc. Fresh fruit has the most fiber and the least amount of sugar. If you do choose dried fruits, read the ingredients to make sure there is no added sugar or sulfites. If you choose juices, then make sure there is no added sugar. When choosing fruits and vegetables, look up the 12 most toxic and 12 least toxic list. If you cannot afford organic, then avoid the 12 most toxic and eat from the 12 least toxic (or choose the 12 most toxic to be the only organic ones to buy).

Drinks:

- Drinks to limit: Soda, sweetened ice tea drinks (Arizona, Lipton, Snapple), sweetened fruit drinks (Ocean Spray, Crystal Light, Kool-Aid, PowerAde, Gatorade, etc.) energy drinks (Red Bull, Monster, etc.) and cocoas/hot chocolate/ chocolate milk/flavored milk. Many drinks that claim to be "healthy herbal" drinks are also very sweetened. Remember, READ LABELS, even on your beverages.

- Drinks that are acceptable: water; unsweetened fruit juices (no more than 6 – 8 oz./day, and you can dilute with water to make 12 – 16 oz./day; unlimited veggie juices (low salt V-8, tomato juice or fresh s?ueezed veggie juice; do no over do it on the carrot and beet juices because they have a higher sugar content); cow/goat/soy/rice/almond/oat milk (check ingredients to make sure there is no added sugar); herbal and Green tea (that you steep yourself; if you cannot have caffeine then do not drink Green tea); plain sparkling mineral waters/club soda/ seltzer water/ (add lemon juice or a splash of fruit juice to it for a better flavor); and Coffee substitutes. A great drink is mineral water with added Stevia flavors (such as vanilla, root beer, or chocolate raspberry). They are very refreshing, and satisfy any soda cravings.
- Water: Drink at least . your weight in ounces of water per day. For every caffeinated drink, add an extra 8oz. of water per day.
- Coffee: Limit to 1 – 2 cups per day (this is up to you. If coffee is one thing you cannot live without, just make sure you are drinking enough water to keep hydrated =. your weight in ounces + an extra 8oz. for every 8oz. of caffeinated beverage). If you are sensitive to caffeine or cannot have it for other reasons, you may try coffee substitutes such as, Caffix, Pero, Teechino, and Roma. It is best to drink coffee/coffee substitutes black or with added milk, but no sugar. A sweetener substitute that is good to add to coffee is li?uid Stevia. Whole Foods and Sprouts has many flavors, such as regular, French vanilla, dark chocolate, strawberry, etc. They are located in the medicinal herb section of Whole Foods and Sprouts. Other stores may have Stevia, but not as many options

(see section on sugar below for more information on Stevia).

Sugars:

- Negative effects of sugar: Sugar depresses the immune system for up to 5 hours eating it. It is a major source of inflammation in our bodies. It causes imbalances in blood sugar level, and can lead to diabetes when consumed in large quantities on a regular basis. Considered to be one of the factors n severe cases of PMS in women.
- LIMIT AS MUCH AS POSSIBLE (OR JUST AVOID): WHITE AND BROWN SUGAR, HONEY, AND ARTIFICIAL SWEETENERS (INCLUDING SPLENDA). Honey should be used sparingly, because it is sugar (just in a natural form). Other names that white sugar goes by on labels: sucrose, glucose, fructose, dextrose, maltose, corn syrup solids, and high fructose corn syrup solids. Stay away from corn syrup of any kind. Watch out for hidden sugars. Most low fat and non – fat foods are high sugars. READ YOUR LABELS, and you will do fine.
- Glycemic index – The glycemic index explains the difference between different carbohydrates by ranking carbs according to their effect on our

blood sugar levels.

- Choosing low glycemic carbs – the ones that produce only small fluctuations in our blood sugar and insulin levels – helps by reducing your risk of heart disease and diabetes and is the key to sustainable weight loss. A website you can use to look up the glycemic index on food is: http://www.glycemicindex.com/.

- Stevia: Stevia is a sweetener that I prefer for my drinks. It can also be used on food. Stevia is an herb that is about 3000 times sweeter than sugar (remember this is when adding to food). It's a natural sweetener, and does not add any sugar or calories to your food. A brand that I like is Sweet Leaf liquid stevia. It comes in regular flavor, and a variety of other flavors, such as French, chocolate, toffee nut, chocolate raspberry, lemon drop, and root beer. People have even used this to sweeten homemade ice cream to make a healthier treat. Be careful when adding at first, and do just a little at a time. If you over do the Stevia it can actually have a bitter taste. Some people do not like the taste of Stevia at all, because it is different from sugar, but if you are looking for a sweetener alternative, it is worth trying. It tastes a little different than sugar, but it can satisfy a sweet tooth.

- Other sweet options are: fruit, unsweetened fruit juice, a small serving of unsweetened dry fruit (raisins, dates, cranberries, etc.) all-fruit jams, all-fruit syrups, or 100% Maple Syrup. I would still limit these to one serving per day (check serving size on jams and syrups) except for Maple syrup (which is better used less often due to high sugar content like honey).

- Substitute sweeteners for baking are: un-sulfured blackstrap molasses; blue agave syrup; date sugar; Mystic Lake Fruit Concentrate and/or Fruitsource (pineapple syrup); Brown Rice Syrup; Malted Barley Syrup. These are great to help lower the sugar content in your baked goods, so when you do eat sweet things, they are still healthier.

- Blue agave syrup is another sweetener option that is natural and low on the glycemic index. You can find this at most health food stores or in the healthy aisles of grocery stores like Fry's (Smiths).

- Sweet tooth: If you have a big sweet tooth, I find it best to have 1- 2 days a week where you allow yourself to have one normal sized treat, so you do not end up binging on junk food down the road.

SEVEN

DO'S AND DON'TS

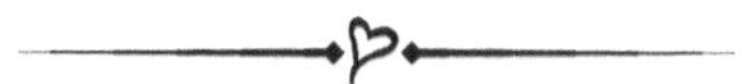

Do's

- Follow the diet and instructions accordingly.

- List all medications prescribed to you by your personal physician in the medical health history packet.

- Drink a minimum of 1/2 gallon of bottled/filtered water and/or unsweetened tea daily.

- Light exercise (walking 20-30 minutes is allowed).

- Get some sun. Studies show that daily sunshine exposure on your skin can increase your Vitamin D blood levels.

- Vitamin D deficiency can put you at risk for certain cancers. In?uire about ordering the Vitamin D 25-hydroxy serum blood test.

- Use food seasonings to flavor food but read labels to avoid sugar, starches, or sugar alcohols.

- Use a Natural Sweetener. Stevia is recommended during the HCG diet. Please avoid artificial sweeteners such as Splenda, E?ual, and Sweet 'N Low.

- Eat grapefruit. Grapefruit has been scientifically proven to release fat.

- Eat 3-5 times per day. This improves your metabolism and helps release excess fat reserves.

- Try to eat organically (meat, fruits, and vegetables). Organic food does not contain preservatives, chemicals, flavor enhancers, herbicides, pesticides, growth hormones, or antibiotics, which are known to cause illness or potential weight gain. If organic food is not accessible, look for chicken products in your local supermarket that do not contain antibiotics; fish products that are not farm raised and only wild-caught;

and wash all fruits and vegetables thoroughly.

- Add Fiber. Fiber helps to relieve constipation, reduce appetite, improve digestion, and cleanse the body of micro-toxins.

Don'ts

- Don't use products containing oil, such as lotions, make-up, and cream on skin or scalp.
- Eliminate carbonated beverages. They can interfere with calcium absorption, causing nutritional deficiencies and slowing down the digestion.
- Do not make changes or substitutions to the diet, even if they contain fewer calories. This will negatively interfere with the program.
- Don't use fats. This includes oil and margarine in cooking, or ingesting fats in any form.
- Don't eat sugar or chew gum.
- Avoid sugar-free foods and foods with known starches.
- Avoid all sweets and dairy products.
- No MSG (Monosodium Glutamate).
- No Fast Food.
- No Fried Food.
- No added Salt.

Disclaimer

Introduction

By using this book, you accept this disclaimer in full.

No advice

The book contains information. The information is not advice and should not be treated as such.

No representations or warranties

To the maximum extent permitted by applicable law and subject to section below, we exclude all representations, warranties, undertakings and guarantees relating to the book.

Without prejudice to the generality of the foregoing paragraph, we do not represent, warrant, undertake or guarantee:

- that the information in the book is correct, accurate, complete or non-misleading.

- that the use of the guidance in the book will lead to any particular outcome or result.

Limitations and exclusions of liability

The limitations and exclusions of liability set out in this section and elsewhere in this disclaimer: are subject to section 6 below; and govern all liabilities arising under the disclaimer or in relation to the book, including liabilities arising in contract, in tort (including negligence) and for breach of statutory duty.

We will not be liable to you in respect of any losses arising out of any event or events beyond our reasonable control.

We will not be liable to you in respect of any business losses, including without limitation loss of or damage to profits, income, revenue, use, production, anticipated savings, business, contracts, commercial opportunities or goodwill.

We will not be liable to you in respect of any loss or corruption of any data, database or software.

We will not be liable to you in respect of any special, indirect or consequential loss or damage.

Exceptions

Nothing in this disclaimer shall: limit or exclude our liability for death or personal injury resulting from negligence; limit or exclude our liability for fraud or fraudulent misrepresentation; limit any of our liabilities in any way that is not permitted under applicable law; or exclude any of our liabilities that may not be excluded under applicable law.

Severability

If a section of this disclaimer is determined by any court or other competent authority to be unlawful and/or unenforceable, the other sections of this disclaimer continue in effect.

If any unlawful and/or unenforceable section would be lawful or enforceable if part of it were deleted, that part will be deemed to be deleted, and the rest of the section will continue in effect.

Law and jurisdiction

This disclaimer will be governed by and construed in accordance with Swiss law, and any disputes relating to this disclaimer will be subject to the exclusive jurisdiction of the courts of Switzerland.